A GUIDE TO YOUR PREGNANCY

A GUIDE TO YOUR PREGNANCY

Simple a nswers to your complex questions

MANOJ PAPRIKAR

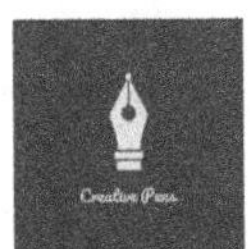

Published by Manoj Paprikar
Madhu-Mukund, Plot no. 6, Sector C, Nausha Ganpati,
Gangapur road, Nashik, 422005
Published in Nashik, India

Printed and bound by Notion Press
Old No.38, New No. 6, McNichols Road, Chetpet
Chennai-600031

This edition published August 2019

ISBN 9789353826079
Copyright © Manoj Paprikar 2019

Cover Photo : Alicia Petresc from Unsplash.com : Creative common license

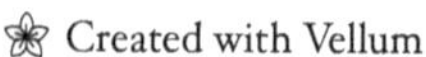 Created with Vellum

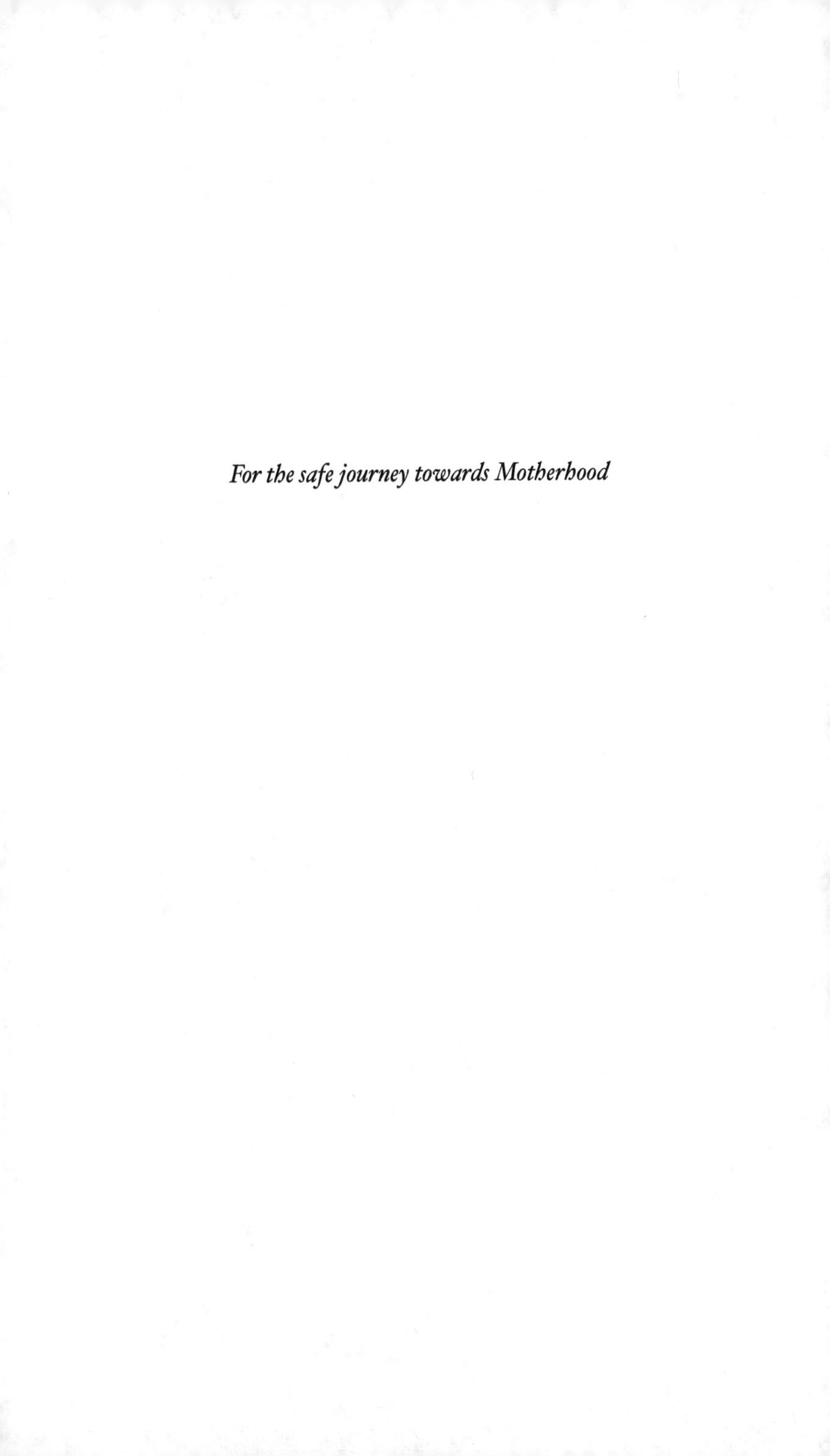

For the safe journey towards Motherhood

CONTENTS

FOREWORD

Pregnancy is a physiological condition. This simple fact is lost on most of the patients who seek consultation for Antenatal care. After working in this field as a gynaecologist for almost thirteen years, I felt the need to write this book which drives home this same point.

Most patients are unaware or lack basic knowledge about this physiological journey which they have decided to undertake, with the hope of bringing in a new life into this world. Blame it on the education or lack of proper guidance, the fact remains that they are ill informed and not prepared for this journey. They have to have correct, simple and scientific information to guide them in this process.

In this age of information overload, there is no dearth of educational material on the internet. But gaining that knowledge and putting it into proper perspective needs some guidance and medical consultation. Otherwise, it adds to the anxiety and burden of the woman.

The traditional source of this information has been the joint and extended families. The senior and experienced ladies handing out correct, rational and sometimes prejudiced information to the mother in question. But, this family system has broken down due to small and nuclear families. The couple may not be privy to this knowledge readily. Hence, it is pertinent that the mother or the couple have a reliable and simple to follow source of information.

Any resource on pregnancy management is no substitute for a medical consultation . But understanding the normal physiology, the expected bodily changes and danger signals is of utmost importance. If the couple is well conditioned and informed of these anticipated milestones, then the adaptation and acceptance of the journey is much more smooth, pleasurable and enjoyable for them.

The concept of writing this book is the same. Make the couple understand the basic physiology. The expected changes. The remedial solutions. And most importantly, watch for the danger signals.

This book has been written with this concept in mind for making the motherhood a journey to be cherished, enjoyed and definitely safe.

Dr. Manoj Paprikar M.S. (Obs & Gyn)
08 Aug 2019

CHAPTER 1
PRE CONCEPTIONAL COUNSELLING

WHAT IS PRE-CONCEPTIONAL COUNSELLING

It is the counselling done before the pregnancy with the aim of identifying any problem areas which can be addressed.

Centre for Disease Control (CDC) defines it as

"A set of interventions that aim to identify and modify biomedical, behavioural, and social risks to a woman's health or pregnancy outcome through prevention and management."

WHEN SHOULD I TAKE IT?

It should be planned when you are contemplating pregnancy. It would involve a visit to your doctor and certain tests.It should be done at least six months in advance, so that you can take corrective action if required.

BENEFITS OF PRE-CONCEPTIONAL COUNSELLING

It prepares you for the journey towards motherhood. It is

the first step and helps you to embark on this journey in a positive, confident and educated way.

The benefits are listed below.

1. It improves knowledge, attitude and preparedness of the couple.
2. Baseline tests are performed to know the general well being of the lady.
3. Identifies any major medical illnesses like Diabetes, Hypertension, Hypothyroidism etc
4. Corrective action can be taken to control the diseases so as to get an optimal outcome in the pregnancy.
5. Helps in minimising pregnancy losses.
6. It helps in screening for genetic conditions in the family and creates an awareness about it. Remedial action for the same can be taken if required.

CHRONIC MEDICAL CONDITIONS

Many medical conditions can affect pregnancy. Most of them will have some bearing on the pregnancy. But certain conditions are very common and may be missed if they are not checked for. Following conditions are therefore routinely checked.

DIABETES MELLITUS

Uncontrolled Diabetes in the pregnant mother complicates pregnancy in a number of ways. The following adverse effects are well known:

- Anomalies in the baby like Neural tube defects.
- Big size baby leading to problems during delivery.

• Sudden intra uterine fetal demise.

Hence, it is very important that pre existing Diabetes be diagnosed and controlled if the lady wants to go in for a pregnancy.

Blood sugar levels, Urine examination and Glycosylated Haemoglobin levels are used to identify Diabetes. An optimum control of sugar should be ascertained before planning the pregnancy.

HYPERTENSION

Hypertension which is present before the lady gets pregnant is called Essential hypertension. Such hypertension should be optimally managed with suitable therapy like lifestyle modification, exercise, diet and drugs. The patient should also undergo tests to know the extent of damage caused by hypertension.

Pregnancy per se can induce hypertension. It is called Pregnancy Induced Hypertension or Pre Eclampsia. It can have a deleterious effect on the baby as well as mother.

So, pre existing hypertension can complicate such pregnancies and pose additional risk to the mother as well as fetus.

THYROID DISORDERS

Thyroid status should be checked in non pregnant state so as to pick up Hyper or Hypo thyroidism. Both the conditions have adverse outcomes. Hypothyroid condition is more common.

The condition is diagnosed by assessing the T3, T4 and TSH levels in the blood.

In case of Hypothyroidism, simple substitution with the

thyroid hormone will solve the problem and prevent untoward effects like impaired development in the baby.

SUBSTANCE ABUSE

Alcohol, nicotine, narcotic or other substance abuses have a deleterious effect on the baby in varied proportions. Mother should be off these drugs before contemplating pregnancy.

EPILEPSY

The risk of having congenital structural anomalies in the babies is high in mothers having epilepsy.

This risk is because of the genetic make up of the mother and also because of anti epileptic medications she may be taking for the same.

Hence, she should be evaluated and if possible the drugs should be stopped or converted to the ones which are least detrimental to the baby.

Usually single drug therapy is better than multi drug therapy.

OBESITY

Obesity has multiple problems in pregnancy. It in itself can lead to labour and delivery difficulties. It can lead to complications during Cesarean delivery.

Obesity also puts the mother at an increased risk of developing Diabetes and Hypertension in pregnancy.

Hence, every effort should be made to make the mother achieve near normal weight before she plans the baby.

. . .

MAJOR MEDICAL DISORDERS

Many medical diseases like Heart disorders, Immunological or Kidney diseases can aggravate the condition of the mother as well as have an adverse effect on the fetus. The would–be mother should be properly evaluated and optimally managed before she decides to plan for pregnancy.

CONGENITAL MALFORMATIONS

There are multiple reasons for having congenital malformations in the baby. Assessing these factors can help in identifying and preventing these malformations in the fetus. They are briefly discussed below.

CHROMOSOMAL DISORDERS

These are due to alteration in the number or characteristics of the chromosomes. A carrier mother or father can affect the baby, or it can be due to a spontaneous occurrence.

Common examples are

- Trisomy 21 (an extra chromosome no. 21 instead of normal two.)
- Trisomy 18
- Trisomy 13

SINGLE GENE DISORDERS

Genes are the building blocks of the DNA. Any alterations or deletions of individual genes will give rise to gene disorders. The defect in the gene will be manifested by some structural, chemical or developmental defect in the body.

These defects in the mother or the father are transmitted via the ova or the sperm. They follow complex transmission patterns. Knowing the exact disorder in the parents can help predict the likelihood of the disease in the offspring.

Examples are

- Cystic fibrosis
- Haemophilia
- Achondroplasia
- Muscular dystrophy

INFECTIONS

Maternal infections like Toxoplasma, Rubella, Cytomegalovirus and Herpes can give rise to congenital abnormalities in the fetus.

MULTIFACTORIAL

An interplay of many factors like genetic predisposition and environmental factors are responsible for some abnormalities.

Common examples are

- Cleft lip/palate
- Congenital heart defects
- Neural tube defects

SO SHOULD I TAKE IT?

Yes, absolutely. If you take it in time, it will ensure that you undertake the journey towards motherhood in a confident, informed and a healthy way.

Take the preconception counselling at least six months in advance to help you understand all the issues and take corrective actions if needed.

CHAPTER 2
DIAGNOSIS OF PREGNANCY

THE NORMAL MENSTRUAL CYCLE

The normal menstrual cycle ranges from 21 to 28 days. The flow lasts anywhere between 3 to 6 days. The cycle is counted from the first day of the Last Menstrual Period. Commonly referred to as L.M.P.

In an exact 28 days cycle, ovulation takes place in the middle of the cycle. *i.e.* day 14. But if the cycle length is more, then the ovulation shifts correspondingly away from the L.M.P.

Putting it the other way, ovulation usually occurs 14 days prior to the next expected period. Hence it cannot be predicted if the cycles are not regular.

The entire cycle is controlled by brain. (Hypothalamus) The hormones affect the ovaries which secrete estrogen and progesterone which in turn have an effect on the uterus.

The endometrium is the inner lining of uterus which is cyclically shed due to this interplay of hormones.

. . .

How are dates calculated ?

Dates are calculated from the Last Menstrual Period. LMP.

Pregnancy duration is 40 weeks or 280 days. Hence it is added to the LMP, to get the expected date of delivery, called EDD.

Hence, if

LMP:01/01/2019

EDD:07/10/2019

Usually Obstetricians wait till the EDD for spontaneous onset of labour pains, if everything is normal. An early intervention is done if there are any problems like reduced liquor, decreased fetal movements or pregnancy induced hypertension.

How is pregnancy diagnosed?

The most common test which is used to diagnose pregnancy is the Urine Pregnancy Test. (UPT) or the Gravindex test.

It detects the levels of hormone called HCG (Human Chorionic Gonadotropin) in urine of the patient. This test is very accurate and is rarely wrong.

It will detect the pregnancy at about 20-22 days from the LMP. That means it can become positive even if the patient has not missed her periods.

So, UPT is the first test that becomes positive. It is the most common and reliable test for diagnosing pregnancy.

What is Missing the periods ?

The most important effect of conception is cessation of menses. So you will miss the period in case of a pregnancy.

The periods will not commence on the expected date. So, any missed periods should raise the suspicion of pregnancy.

It is also called Amenorrhoea.

WHY DOES IT OCCUR?

The answer is because of the raised level of progesterone hormone which is secreted by the pregnancy. Normally, during the normal menstrual cycle, there is a dip in both estrogen and progesterone which causes the menses. Now because of pregnancy, this does not occur. The endometrium is required for the continuation of the pregnancy.

WHAT IS BETA HCG? IS IT ALWAYS REQUIRED?

No. Beta HCG (Human Chorionic Gonadotropin) is not required in all the cases. It has got select importance and should be done only on the advice of a doctor.

Normally, HCG levels in urine are detected by a Urine pregnancy test. But sometimes we need to know the exact levels of HCG in blood. Beta HCG levels tell us that.

It is done in certain problematic conditions like ectopic or molar pregnancy.

WHEN IS FIRST ULTRA SONOGRAPHY DONE?

USG or Ultra Sonography is done usually at 6 weeks of pregnancy. Why is it done? Well, the answer is simple.

For knowing the location, size, number and viability of the pregnancy.

IS IT DONE ABDOMINALLY OR INTERNALLY?

Usually earlier on, before seven weeks, it is done using a vaginal route.

Later on, it is done abdominally, as the pregnancy can be seen from above.

IS IT SAFE?

Yes, it is absolutely safe. In the current strength and dose of the ultrasound (Sound Energy) it is very safe. It has no effect on the small baby.

WHAT ARE THE BASIC TESTS THAT I NEED TO TAKE?

There is a set protocol for doing the basic tests during the pregnancy as per standard guidelines.

The following tests are routinely done:

1. Complete Blood counts
2. Blood sugar levels
3. Thyroid hormone levels
4. Viral markers for Hepatitis, HIV and Syphilis
5. Urine examination

Apart from these basic tests certain other tests may be prescribed by the doctor as per requirement; especially if there is any high risk to the pregnancy or any pre existing medical condition.

WHAT ARE THE WARNING SIGNS I SHOULD BE AWARE OF?

The most important problem is that of abortion. Early pregnancy is at an important risk of getting aborted.

It should be kept in mind that almost 30-40 percent pregnancies are aborted. It is the law of nature. Most of the times the factors are genetic in nature. We have no control over it.

As the pregnancy advances and the fetal heart beat is seen on USG, the chances of abortion decrease.

CHAPTER 3

PHYSIOLOGICAL CHANGES OF PREGNANCY

It is very important that the pregnant woman understands the changes that will normally take place in the course of her pregnancy. If she knows what is normal and what to expect, she can cope up with it in a better way.

It goes without saying that she will understand the normal changes that are expected and what is abnormal. It will allay her fear and anxiety.

This chapter discusses the common and important changes that are normal in pregnancy.

CHANGES IN GENITAL ORGANS

Uterus

The uterus increases massively in size from a mere 60 gm to about a kg in weight. The length increases from 7.5 cm to about 35 cm.

The uterus reaches the umbilicus by about 6 months and the tip of the abdominal cavity-xiphisternum by 36 weeks.

Vagina

The vulva and the vagina become edematous and vascular. The increased blood supply causes a bluish discolouration of the vaginal walls, called as Jacquemier's sign.

The secretions become thick, whitish and copious. The pH also drops becoming more acidic. It is due to the effect of Lactobacillus under the effect of Estrogen. It has a protective effect.

Too much of douching and frequent use of vaginal washes is not advisable as it may disturb the normal balance of the vaginal bacterial flora.

Unless associated with itching, bleeding and a confirmed infection, mild vaginal discharge does not require any treatment.

BREAST CHANGES

The breasts gradually increase in size under the influence of both Estrogen and Progesterone. This is due to hypertrophy, proliferation and secretory changes in the alveoli of the breast.

There may be enlargement and pain in the axillary area, which is due to an extension of the mammary tissue in the axilla. It is usually because of rudimentary breast tissue. But it can raise an alarm due to the sudden increase in size.

The breast starts secreting milk in the form of colostrum as early as 12th week. It can be squeezed out of the nipples and is perfectly normal.

SKIN CHANGES

Chloasma or mask of pregnancy

It is the hyperpigmentation that is observed on the face. It is hormonally mediated and is normal. It usually wears off after pregnancy

Linea Nigra

It is a linear black marking which appears on the midline of the abdomen. It is due to a hormone called MSH. (Melanocyte Stimulating Hormone)

It is normal and the effect usually wears off after pregnancy.

Striae Gravidarum

These are light pink marks on the skin found on the abdomen and extending on the thighs and even on to the breasts. They turn white after the delivery and are then called striae albicans.

Massage and use of oil to a certain extent reduces them. They are benign and can't be totally prevented.

WEIGHT GAIN IN PREGNANCY

The average weight gain in pregnancy is 10-12 kgs. Approximate weight gain is as follows:

Ist trimester :1kg

IInd Trimester:5 kg

IIIrd Trimester:5 kg

The fetus, placenta, liquor, uterus and breasts constitute about 6 kg gain. The rest of the 6 kg is due to maternal gain due to fat, protein, blood and fluid increase.

The average extra caloric requirement of the mother is only 500 kcal over and above her normal requirement.

OBESITY

Obese patients should not attempt to lose weight in pregnancy. They should restrict unnecessary weight gain. Weight gain should be about 7 to 8 kgs only.

CHANGES IN BLOOD

Blood Volume

The amount of fluid that is gained during pregnancy is about 6.5 litres, about half of which contributes towards the fetus.

Pregnancy is a state of hypervolemia as there is retention of fluid, sodium and potassium. There is an increase in blood volume by about 40-50 %.

HAEMOGLOBIN

The Red Blood Cell mass rises by about 20-30 % which is less than plasma volume increase. So there is a lag as compared to the plasma volume. Hence blood is diluted.

The Hb percentage drops by about 2 gm and the Haematocrit by 15-20%.

These changes are physiological and serve to help the pregnancy. But excessive drop or deficit is not good, hence iron supplementation is required during the course of pregnancy.

JOINTS AND LIGAMENTS

The ligaments become lax and supple due to the effect of hormones and fluid retention. This is to facilitate the relaxation of the pelvis, so that the baby easily passes through the pelvis during labor.

The most important effect is back-pain and joint aches.

Back-pain is common as there is change in posture during the third trimester and hence a change in centre of gravity. It results in excessive strain and hence pain. Massage, oil and relaxant liniments are helpful.

The joints also ache for the same reason. Pain in hands

and fingers is common due to a condition called Carpal Tunnel Syndrome. This is due to pressure on the nerves as they pass under a band over the wrist joint. Hot water fomentation, exercise and vitamins alleviate the problem.

AIR HUNGER

There is a central effect of progesterone on the brain centre. Additionally it makes the respiratory muscles lax and the lady has to breathe more forcefully to satisfy the requirements of the baby.

In addition, the uterus and the baby push up the diaphragm causing more discomfort and decrease in the lung capacity.

All these effects give rise to breathing discomfort, shortness of breath or sometimes air hunger.

All these are normal changes and they are not a cause for concern.

BODY EDEMA OR SWELLING

Due to the fluid retention there is an increase in blood volume and extra cellular fluid. This causes some amount of edema and bloating. It is normal.

Additionally, the fetus also presses on the internal blood vessels and impedes the returning blood to heart. It causes pedal edema. The lady should take walks regularly and take a pillow under her feet while sleeping.

If the blood pressure is normal and the edema is minimal, it is not a cause of worry. If B.P. also rises then it becomes more worrisome and should be addressed at the earliest.

CHAPTER 4

THE FIRST TRIMESTER

NAUSEA AND VOMITING OF PREGNANCY

Nausea and vomiting of pregnancy is the most common problem and complaint during the first three months of pregnancy. It usually starts around six weeks and peaks around ten to twelve weeks. Thereafter it subsides gradually.

WHY DOES IT OCCUR?

It is because of the raised levels of circulating HCG in the blood. It is in a way welcome, because it signifies that the pregnancy is doing fine.

Severe form is controlled using dietary modifications and medicines.

HOW TO PREVENT IT?

The best way of preventing is to avoid oily, pungent, spicy

food with strong flavours and smell. That triggers the centre in the brain for vomiting.

The food should be light, nutritious, balanced and fresh. It should include fresh fruits, vegetables, sprouts and salads.

It is advisable to eat three major meals and three small snacks. It is better to eat in small portions and more frequently.

Antacids and anti-emetics should be the last resort and should be taken under medical guidance.

DIET IN PREGNANCY

The most important concept of diet in pregnancy is very simple. Keep your diet balanced. Most of the problems are addressed by a balanced diet.

Indian diet is a perfect balance of carbohydrates, fats and proteins. It is important that this proportion is maintained.

DIETARY PROPORTIONS

50 % carbohydrates, 30 % proteins and 20 % fats. This is the ideal ratio in diet. This ideal proportion should also include adequate roughage or fibre.

Diet should include some amount of multi-grains and bran.

FIBRE IN DIET

The diet should include judicious amounts of salads. They add volume to the diet which prevents constipation and also contribute to vitamins.

Vitamins are required for all the metabolic requirements of the body and their requirement goes up in pregnancy.

· · ·

Fruits

Fruits are also a major contributors of vitamins and anti-oxidants in the diet. They help metabolism and prevent untoward side effects due to the accumulation of toxic radicals.

Citrus fruits like oranges are rich in fibre and should be preferred. Fruits like bananas and apples can significantly increase the blood sugar levels due to high carbohydrate content.

Frequency and Portions

It is preferable that the pregnant lady has three major meals and three small meals. Breakfast, lunch and dinner interspersed with small snacks is the ideal way to have food.

The portions can be small and more frequent. This helps in balancing out the rise in blood sugar levels. Blood sugar levels do not rise to extreme levels, which is more detrimental to the baby.

Dietary supplements

If the diet is wholesome and nutritious, then there is no need for taking unnecessary food supplements.

The only scientifically recommended supplement is Folic Acid, which must be taken. Deficiency of Folic acid is known to cause congenital defects in the baby like Neural tube defects.

Apart from this other vitamins and food supplements are not required if the diet is complete and wholesome.

TRAVELLING DURING FIRST TRIMESTER

Most patients ask me this question. Can I travel? Can I use

four wheeler to drive to my work place? Well, the answer is simple.

It is better to avoid unnecessary travel, especially by road. If at all you have to travel, use a four wheeler. Bikes and scooters should be totally avoided.

CAN I TRAVEL BY AIR OR BY RAIL?

It is safe to travel by rail, as it is much smoother as compared to travelling by road.

Travelling by air is also very safe, and should be the preferable mode of transport if you have to travel long distances.

CAN I HAVE INTERCOURSE?

Intercourse is not an absolute no–no in pregnancy. But there is a caveat to it.

Rough sex should be avoided as it can induce abortions. So it is better to be gentle and cautious.

Sexual intercourse can lead to infections due to the exchange of body fluids. Barrier method in the form of condoms should be used to prevent it.

FREQUENCY OF VISITS

How frequently should I see my doctor? That's the most common question asked. Well, for the first visit it should be as soon as possible.

First visit is important for ascertaining and diagnosing the pregnancy. All the tests which are done, form the base line against which further changes are compared.

Subsequently, the visits are monthly in the first two trimesters, if everything is normal. The doctor may ask for more visits if problems are identified or the risk is high.

FIRST TRIMESTER ULTRASOUND

First trimester ultrasound is done at 11-13 weeks period of gestation. It involves three parameters as described below.

NUCHAL TRANSLUCENCY

It is the measurement of a translucent area in the posterior part of fetal neck. A raised thickness is associated with chromosomal disorders - aneuploidies. It is an aberration in the number of chromosomes.

The most common being Chromosome 21 and 18. Trisomy 21 is called Down's syndrome and is associated with multiple anomalies and mental retardation.

NASAL BONE

Presence or absence of Nasal bone is checked on ultrasound. Absent nasal bone is a known risk factor for Down's syndrome.

DOUBLE MARKER

Two serum markers are measured - PAPP A and HCG. The levels of these two analytes are combined with Nasal Translucency measurements. It gives a statistical estimate of having Down's syndrome in the baby. It is not a confirmatory test. It gives detection of Down's syndrome in 80% of cases.

FIRST TRIMESTER FETAL ANOMALY DETECTION

The scan of performing NT and NB is utilised for detecting early fetal anomalies. Many anomalies are being picked up with this scan.

However, many anomalies are detected only later in second trimester. Hence it does not substitute the standard Anomaly scan performed after 18 weeks.

CHORIONIC VILLUS SAMPLING (CVS)

Certain genetic conditions are lethal and dangerous. They may recur in subsequent pregnancies. When such conditions are likely, a sample of fetal tissue is obtained and studied in the laboratory.

The chorionic tissue is obtained by using a needle under Ultrasonographic guidance. A very small portion of the tissue is extracted out.

The tissue is subjected to Chromosomal or Gene studies as indicated.

Is there a risk for my baby?

Yes, a small amount of risk due to the surgical procedure is involved. It can be in the form of bleeding, abortion or infection.

But with modern methods and expertise it is not very high. The risk of having a problematic baby must be weighed against the risk of the procedure.

WARNING SYMPTOMS

There are certain symptoms which the pregnant lady must be very careful about. In case of any of these problems, she should immediately report to her treating doctor.

Bleeding

In certain conditions like abortions, bleeding is a warning

symptom. So it should not be taken lightly. It can be a Threatened Abortion.

Other problems leading to bleeding include Molar and Ectopic pregnancy. They require to be evaluated by your doctor.

Pain

Pain can be a warning symptom of Ectopic pregnancy or Abortion.

Other non pregnancy related conditions can also present with pain. e.g. urinary tract infection, renal stone or appendicitis.

Severe Nausea and Vomiting

If there is severe nausea and vomiting, it can lead to severe dehydration and electrolyte imbalance. Such type of patients require hospitalisation and intravenous fluids and medications.

So, if there is a moderate amount of vomiting not responding to medications, immediately consult your doctor and consider hospitalisation.

CHAPTER 5

THE SECOND TRIMESTER

FREQUENCY OF VISITS

The second trimester visits are usually once every four weeks till 28 weeks. Thereafter the visits are increased to once every two weeks till 36 weeks period of gestation.

The frequency can sometimes be increased if there are certain high risk factors like Diabetes or Pregnancy Induced Hypertension.

ANOMALY SCAN

Anomaly scan is also referred to as a level II scan. It is done by a trained Radiologist on a good resolution ultrasonography machine.

The ideal time is at 18-19 weeks of pregnancy. This maximises the chances of picking up any structural defects in the baby.

It should also be remembered that not all small anomalies can be identified on an ultrasound examination.

A timely action can be taken as per the MTP act in case any severe anomaly is identified. As per law MTP is permitted only unto 20 weeks period of gestation in India.

TRIPLE/QUADRUPLE MARKER

It is a hormonal test for either three/ four markers in the blood of the mother. Based on the results a risk estimate is obtained for certain conditions in the baby as mentioned below.

1. Trisomy 21 : Down's syndrome
2. Trisomy 18 : Edward's syndrome
3. Neural tube defects : e.g. spina bifida, anencephaly

It should be kept in mind that these are screening tests. It only gives a statistical estimate(chances) for having one of these conditions in the baby.

The only way to confirm the condition is to go in for Amniocentesis.

WHAT IS AMNIOCENTESIS?

In Amniocentesis, a small needle is poked inside the uterus and small amount of amniotic fluid (baby's water) is drawn out. It contains the chromosomes of the baby. They are studied by performing a Karyotyping. It confirms the chromosomal problems of Trisomy 21/18.

Neural tube defects are identified by Anomaly scans.

It should be kept in mind that Gene disorders are not studied by Karyotyping. Detailed studies are required for it. The treating Obstetrician will guide you if warranted.

SHORT CERVIX

It is also called cervical incompetence. The cervix is apparently loose and cannot hold the baby in position and opens up. This leads to a premature delivery.

A baby born at less than 28 to 30 weeks period of gestation cannot survive in a normal setup. Hence to prevent this, the cervix is given physical support.

Clinical examination and Ultrasound is used to identify it. A cervical length of 2.5 to 3 cm is considered safe.

The doctor takes a decision to put a stitch based on the findings. A prior history of such abortions is a very strong indication for cervical encirclage.

A cervical encirclage or os tightening is performed in Operation theatre under anaesthesia.

BLOOD SUGAR MONITORING

Blood sugar levels are checked in the second trimester because pregnancy makes the mother prone for diabetes. Pregnancy is a diabetogenic state. Hence it is again re evaluated.

The testing is done at about 24 weeks of gestation. It is a two step process.

GLUCOSE CHALLENGE TEST (GCT)

It is a screening test and is done for everyone at 24 to 26 weeks. One need not be fasting for this test.

50 gm of Glucose is given to the mother and blood sugar level is estimated after one hour. A value more than 140 mg % is considered abnormal.

Further testing is done for a raised value.

. . .

Glucose Tolerence Test (GTT)

This test involves administering 100 gm of glucose and estimation of four blood sugar levels at 0, 1, 2 and 3 hours.

The test can also be performed by using 75 gm and noting three readings.

If two or more values are abnormal the patient is said to have Gestational Diabetes. Then patient is put on appropriate therapy. It may involve diabetic diet, drugs or even insulin preparations.

BLOOD PRESSURE MONITORING

B.P. monitoring is done at every Antenatal clinic visit. In the second trimester, it is once every two weeks. It would be done more frequently if the B.P. is found to be on a higher side and warrants close monitoring.

Pre Eclampsia

Pre Eclampsia (also called Pregnancy Induced Hypertension) is a condition associated with raised B.P. which is due to pregnancy and starts in the second trimester of pregnancy. It is associated with loss of proteins in the urine. It has multiple detrimental effects on the baby as well as the mother.

The baby suffers with following problems:

Growth restriction

Fetal demise

Abruptio placenta

Fetal death

The mother too is at risk and the condition can deteriorate very rapidly. The baby needs to be delivered early if the mother's life is endangered. The common risks involved are:

Eclampsia or convulsions

Loss of vision

Stroke or brain haemorrhage

Antepartum haemorrhage

ECLAMPSIA

It is the most dreaded complication of Pregnancy induced hypertension. It is a convulsion or fit which the mother throws due to brain edema.

It can be lethal to the baby as well as the mother. It is an emergency and has to be promptly handled.

TRAVELLING

Travelling during second trimester is reasonably safe. It is in fact the best time to travel, if it is a must. Avoiding travel is the best thing to do, but this is the most comfortable time if one can't escape it.

As in first trimester, travel by air is best. As it involves least amount of time. But long distance travel involving more than four or five hours should be preferably avoided. There is risk of blood clotting in the legs due to prolonged immobility. If you undertake such a journey then it is advisable to use compression stalkings and take periodic walks in the aircraft.

Rail journeys are comfortable as compared to road journeys. They offer space for movement and less jerks.

Long distance road journeys should be totally avoided.

EXERCISE IN PREGNANCY

The most common dilemma facing a would be mother is whether to exercise or not. The common advice given by friends and relatives is often conflicting - ranging from resting and not doing anything to taking exercise classes and actively trying to become fit.

Hence, it is wise to spare some time and see what should be ideally and practically done. The following points should clear all the doubts.

It goes without saying that pregnancy, delivery and labor are very physically intense and challenging experiences for the mother. If she goes into it with a physically fit body, that is the best possible thing.

But, at the same time trying to start physical fitness drive, if one is not accustomed to exercise, is also not desirable. What is required is a balanced approach.Best of both the things.

WHEN TO START?

It is best started in the second trimester. By this time you will become more or less free from nausea and vomiting of pregnancy. The general comfort level will also be better now. Hence this is the best time to start physical activity.

HOW MUCH DO I NEED TO EXERCISE?

The thumb rule is that you should exercise about 45 min in a day, at least five times a week. That should suffice.

One can break the duration in multiple spells and increase the overall duration of exercise.

WHAT SHOULD I DO? CARDIO OR STRENGTH?

Well ideally, it should be the combination of both - in equal measures. Cardio improves the stamina of the body and makes it more amenable to withstand prolonged stress of labour . And strength training improves the tone and strength of the muscles. It helps in the labouring process and generating effective bearing down efforts.

. . .

CARDIO TRAINING

The most simple and effective form is taking brisk walks. They are safe, enjoyable and relaxing. Two spells of 30 min each in a day should be enough.

Other exercises could include cycling, swimming and dancing. It should be remembered that all these activities should be done in moderation and not aggressively. Too many jerks are not welcome.

STRENGTH TRAINING

Strength training includes three main components. They are:

Improving the tone of abdominal muscles

Spinal muscle strength

Limbs and pelvic musculature exercises

All the exercises can be performed either using small weights or can be performed in gym by using mechanical training aids.

Most exercises should be done in 8-10 sets and 2 repetitions. A trainer to guide in the exercises is ideal. Following are the samples of exercises which should be performed:

- Dumb bell row
- Pull ups
- Side raise
- Biceps Curl
- Ball squat
- Leg extension
- Pelvic tilt

YOGA

Using yogic breathing exercises like *Pranayam* improve the breathing and lung capacity.

Meditation techniques are very good for decreasing the anxiety and sleep disturbances. It allays fears and helps in staying focused and relaxed.

Yogic exercises in the form of *asanas* are also good for the body. But difficult and dangerous asanas should be completely avoided.

IMMUNISATION

Certain vaccines are routinely administered in pregnancy. Some are given in certain special circumstances.

TETANUS TOXOID (TT)

Two doses of TT are routinely administered in the first pregnancy after 12 weeks of gestation. The two doses should have a gap of one month at least.

If the second or subsequent pregnancy is within five years, only one dose is given the next time.

TETANUS DIPHTHERIA VACCINE (TD)

Combination of Tetanus and Diphtheria is preferred and given in the same dosage schedule.

LEG CRAMPS

Leg cramps usually appear due to the deficiency of Calcium in the blood. Supplementation of calcium in the diet with milk and milk products is beneficial. Calcium should also be taken in the form of tablet or syrup just before meals.

B complex and Vitamin E is also beneficial.

Massage with warm oil and hot water bath is known to help the patients.

CONSTIPATION

The hormonal effect of progesterone and pressure of the growing size of uterus causes constipation.

A diet rich in fibre and green leafy vegetables will benefit. Rice should also be a part of the meals. Plenty of fluids in diet help reducing constipation.

Occasionally constipation may require laxatives to tide over the temporary phase.

CHAPTER 6

THE THIRD TRIMESTER

THIRD TRIMESTER TESTS

Routine antenatal examination forms the bedrock of any assessment. It is supplemented by using the following routine tests:

- Haemogram
- Blood sugar levels
- Urine examination
- Thyroid examination if required

Specialized tests are warranted in high risk cases and other medical disorders. They will be advised by your obstetrician depending upon the situation.

THE GROWTH SCAN

The growth scan is usually performed at 32 weeks period of gestation and repeated at 36 weeks if required.

It helps in assessing the growth of the baby as per expectations. It assesses the fetal well being by studying the fetal biometry(measurements) and the status of liquor amnii. Doppler studies of the fetal blood vessels also give vital additional information.

Any deviation from the normal alerts the doctor and he can take remedial steps. A correction of responsible factor or appropriate treatment is initiated.

FETAL MOVEMENT COUNT

Cardiff Count 10

Patient is supposed to count ten movements starting from 9 a.m. If she perceives it then she can stop counting.

It is abnormal and she has to report back if :

1. there are less than 10 movements in 12 hours on 2 successive days
2. no movements perceived for 12 hours.

DAILY FETAL MOVEMENT COUNT (DFMC)

Patient has to make a note of fetal movements for one hour after each meal. *i.e. Breakfast, Lunch and Dinner.*

She has to multiply counted kicks by four. It gives total kicks in 12 hours. Less than 10 kicks in 12 hours is abnormal. It should raise an alarm and she should consult her doctor.

NON STRESS TEST

A electronic monitoring of fetal heart rate is traced continuously along with the fetal movements. It is something like an ECG.

It alerts us about the fetal well being and the state of

placental adequacy. It assures that the fetus is getting adequate oxygen and is at no immediate risk.

Normal NST is called Reassuring. It is performed after 30 weeks period of gestation and may be repeated every 2-3 weeks.

WARNING SIGNS

There are certain warning signs which need immediate attention. It may also warrant admission to the hospital. Keep these in mind especially in the last trimester.

1. Bleeding from the vagina
2. Gush of fluid from the vagina
3. Severe pains
4. Decreased Fetal movements

BLEEDING FROM VAGINA

Any bleeding in the last trimester can be dangerous. It can be due to various reasons. The most likely cause is onset of labour pains.

Labour Pains

It signifies the onset of labour pains. These pains are associated with intermittent tightening of the uterus accompanied by pain. Initially it comes in about once every 10-15 min and gradually intensifies.It is also associated with a bloody mucoid discharge called as 'Show'.

Placenta Previa

Placenta previa is a condition in which the placenta covers the internal cervical opening. It can be either Complete or Partial.

If it lies in the lower part of the uterus, it is called low lying placenta.

The placenta usually does not actually migrate, as is believed. There is only an apparent shift as the size of uterus increases.

There is a serious risk of haemorrhage in this condition. It is usually painless and sudden. It can become very dangerous and can be recurrent.

Abruptio Placenta

The placenta sometimes prematurely separates from the uterus before the delivery. It is called Placental Abruption.

There can be severe bleeding. Sometimes it can also remain concealed, accumulating inside.

It is usually painful.

It can be potentially fatal for the fetus, if severe.

There is a substantial risk of coagulation disorder. It can pose a serious risk to mother's life as well.

Prompt delivery is undertaken, preferably normally.

GUSH OF FLUID FROM THE VAGINA

The condition results from the rupture of the bag of membranes. The amniotic fluid gushes out and wets the clothes.

It is usually profuse and must not be confused with the mild wetness of the vagina or Candidial curdy discharge.

Rupture of Membranes is usually associated with the onset of Labour. Sometimes Labour pains set in after the ROM. Premature Rupture of Membranes (PROM) is when it occurs prematurely without the patient going into Labor. It can also occur before Term, then called as Preterm PROM.

One should immediately rush to the hospital for admission.

· · ·

SEVERE PAIN

The main cause of severe pain is the onset of Labour. Labour pains are intermittent and associated with tightening of the uterus. They start with about once in every fifteen minutes and will gradually become more frequent.

These pains can be associated with Show or Rupture of Membranes.

DECREASED FETAL MOVEMENTS

Fetal movements are the most important indicator of Fetal well being. They are monitored by various methods. The most commonly used ones are as follows:

1. Daily Fetal Movement Count (DFMC) Fetal movements are counted one hour after each meal; breakfast, lunch and dinner. A total count of ten movements is considered adequate.
2. Cardiff Count to Ten

CHAPTER 7

DELIVERY

WHAT TO EXPECT IN LABOUR

Labour pains are one of the strongest pains that the human body experiences. It ranks second only to dental pain in severity. So yes, Labour is a painful affair and there is no escaping the reality.

But having said this, it is also not true that it is unbearable. With the right frame of mind, adequate mental preparation and knowledge of what to expect, one can surmount the challenge.

There are various techniques and methods available to alleviate the pain and suffering. Modern medicine has made life of a labouring women a bit better.

Following discussion which will answer all your doubts.

LABOUR

Labour is the process of childbirth from the onset of regular uterine contractions until expulsion of the placenta.

It is broadly divided into four stages.

• • •

Stage I

It starts from the onset of labour to the full dilation of cervix. It is again made up of two stages.

Latent Phase

It is more of a preparatory phase of labor in which the connective tissue of cervix changes considerably. The cervix becomes soft and supple. It gets gradually taken up which is also called effacement. In simple words the cervix becomes part of the uterus and it becomes one single passage for the baby to pass through.

The average duration is 8 hours. More in first pregnancies.(Nulliparas) It is said to be prolonged if it's more than 20 in nulliparas and 14 hours in multiparas.

Active phase

Active phase begins after 3 cm of cervical dilation or rupture of membranes.

In Primis it is about 6-8 hours and in multiparas about 4-6 hours.

Stage II

This stage begins from full cervical dilatation and lasts till the the delivery of the baby.

Duration is about 20 to 50 min.

Stage III

This involves the delivery of the placenta and membranes. It can last from about 10 min to an hour.

Sometimes the placenta may fail to separate and require

Manual removal of placenta in Operation Theatre under anaesthesia.

STAGE IV

It is one hour post delivery wherein the patient is observed for all the vital parameters.

POST PARTUM HEMORRHAGE

It is the most dreaded and life threatening complication after the delivery of the baby. It can be unpredictable, unexpected and even prove fatal at times to the mother.

It occurs because of failure of the uterus to contract after the baby is delivered and the placenta expelled out. The uterus—when it contracts, catches the blood vessels in the muscle fibres like a scissors and stops the bleeding. If the uterus for some reasons fails, torrential bleeding results.

Uterine massage and Utero-tonic drugs are given. Sometimes patient may require surgery to stop the bleeding. Sometimes the uterus may be removed to save the mother's life. It is called post-partum hysterectomy.

PSYCHOLOGICAL PREPARATION

A lot is said about the psychological makeup of the patient as it is very important. It makes her prepared for the long arduous journey of labour.

If she is in the right frame of mind and goes forward with positivity she can overcome the challenge very easily and effectively.

Benefits accrue when she is well prepared in the following ways:

- Knowledge of the normal labour process
- Anticipated duration of labour
- Severity of pain
- Advantages of having a normal delivery vis a vis Cesarean section
- A wanted pregnancy
- Family and spouse support
- Emotional and logistic support

CESAREAN SECTION

Cesarean section is a surgical operation performed to deliver the baby through the abdominal wall. It involves an incision on the lower abdomen which cuts the muscle and uterus and delivers the baby.

Advantages

- The most important advantage is that it is fast.
- It is painless as it is done under anaesthesia.
- It does not put the baby under too much of stress as it is fast.
- It cam be life saving for the baby as well as the mother in emergency situations.

DISADVANTAGES

- It is a surgical procedure and has its own set of risks like allergic reaction, bleeding, infection, damage to other structures and residual effects.
- It takes more time for recovery.
- The structural strength never returns to complete normal.

- Chances of repeat Cesarean in next pregnancy is very high.
- It is more expensive.

THE MOST IMPORTANT THING TO REMEMBER IS THAT having a normal delivery is preferable. At the same time, if the situation warrants, there should be no hesitation in going for a Cesarean section if it is in the best interest of the mother and baby. The decision should be left to your treating doctor as he is in the best position to take a decision for you.

LABOUR ANALGESIA

Labour analgesia(pain relief) is the analgesia which is used during the process of Labour. There are different options available. You can choose as per the availability.

Also important is the psychological preparedness of the patient. Counselling and support goes a long way in facing the arduous journey of Labour.

NARCOTIC ANALGESICS

Intra muscular or Intra venous injections are given during the course of Labour, usually Narcotic or its derivatives. They are very potent. They are used in the initial phase of the labour.

Some amount of drug crosses the placenta and can affect the baby. The baby sometimes gets depressed and may have breathing difficulty, but can be readily treated with drugs and usually recovers well.

· · ·

INHALATION ANAESTHETICS

A combination of Oxygen and Nitrous oxide is used called as ETNOX. It is given by mask. Patient breathes and inhales the gaseous mixture through a one way mechanism.

Minimal side effects like nausea, drowsiness and giddiness can occur. It is very safe and patient herself is in control.

EPIDURAL ANAESTHESIA

In this form of anaesthesia, a catheter is placed inside the epidural space. It is frequently topped up with drug to have the desired effect.

The advantage is that the same can be used for performing a Cesarean section. No additional anaesthesia will be required.

Adequate monitoring and availability of Anaesthetist to monitor the patient is a must, and may not be feasible in a busy hospital with inadequate staff.

CHAPTER 8

POST DELIVERY CARE

PUERPERIUM

Puerperium is a period of six weeks following delivery during which the physiological changes that have taken place in the mother, gradually revert back to normal.

Following changes take place which the mother should be aware of. She should know what to expect. And how long it will take.

VAGINA

The vaginal canal will not become like the pre pregnant state. The rugosities will gradually reappear in three to four weeks.

It will regain its natural lubrication and moistness by about six weeks.

UTERUS

Uterus becomes a pelvic organ in two weeks, which means you will not be able to feel it abdominally thereafter. There is no recommendation for using any kind of binders or supports to help in this process. But if you feel comfortable, there is no harm either.

Uterus will go back to its original size in about four weeks.

AFTERPAINS

These are the intermittent pains felt after the delivery. More common in second order or higher pregnancies. Mild pain killers will help in alleviating the pain. It is normal in nature.

STRIAE GRAVIDARUM

These are the markings on the abdomen due to the rupture of the elastic fibres in the skin. They gradually reduce but will not disappear totally.

Oil does not seem to benefit the reduction of striae in a significant way. But its use is not harmful and may only benefit.

ABDOMINAL MUSCLE TONE

The abdominal wall remains soft and flaccid due to the continuous distention that pregnancy had caused. It requires time to regain tone and reach the pre pregnant state.

Exercise will help in regaining the tone. It can be safely started after six weeks.

BREAST FEEDING

Each breast contains 15-20 lobes which in turn are made up of lobules. The small units being alveoli which actually secrete milk. It is drained by the multiple lactiferous ducts directly on the nipple.

WHEN DOES MILK SECRETION START?

It normally starts on first or second day after the delivery. Sometimes mild amount of secretions are noticed in the last months of pregnancy also. It is normal as the breasts are preparing for the final phase under the influence of pregnancy hormones.

COLOSTRUM

It is a deep lemon yellow liquid secreted in the initial stages of breast milk secretion. It contains more minerals, proteins, amino acids and lots of globulin.

Most importantly its constitution is perfectly tailored for the requirements of the baby.

It contains Immunoglobulins (IgA) which gives protection to the baby against infections.

ADVANTAGES OF BREAST FEEDING

It is known to prevent many infections in the baby. It is known to offer protection against allergies, bowel diseases, Diabetes and even Sudden Infant Death syndrome.

So not feeding the baby should be never be a consideration at all, unless advised by doctors.

It is also known that breast fed children have a higher IQ.

Mothers who breast feed have lower risk of breast cancer!

. . .

How to prevent Breast engorgement and Breast fever?

If the baby does not take the feeds timely, there is a chance that the milk forms and accumulates in the breast. It is then very prone to infection.

Moreover, if the nipple hygiene is not proper, and there are cracks on the nipple, then there can be infections. It can later progress even to an abscess, which may require surgical drainage.

Hence timely feeding and keeping the breasts clean and moist is the key to prevent problems.

Do not feed while lying down

It is highly recommended that you feed the baby by taking him in the lap in a proper feeding position. Feeding while sleeping and lying down is dangerous.

The baby can be smothered due to the weight of the breast and may also regurgitate the milk and choke to death. Hence, burping after every feed is also a must.

DEEP VEIN THROMBOSIS

Pregnancy predisposes to clotting of blood due to the effects of hormones. Hence mobilization after the delivery is of paramount importance. Activity should be started as soon as possible. It prevents the stasis of blood and prevents its clotting.

In high risk cases, the doctors will even prescribe anti coagulation drugs to prevent complications.

A dislodged clot from the leg veins can clog the lungs and be fatal. It is called Pulmonary Thromboembolism.

DEPRESSION AND POST PARTUM BLUES

Post part blues are fairly common. It is due to anxiety, fear, excitement, sleep deprivation and various discomforts of pregnancy. If the expectant mother goes into pregnancy with adequate knowledge, it can be minimized.

Usually the Post partum blues are self limiting and will go away with rest, assurance and support from family members.

A severe form exists in the form of Post partum depression. It needs to be identified and treated by consulting psychologist, psychiatrist and medications.

POST DELIVERY CHECK UPS

The first check up after discharge should be ideally after two weeks. And the subsequent visit should be at six weeks after the delivery.

In case of any specific problems the check ups can be more frequent.

Iron and Calcium supplementation should be continued for at least three months post delivery.

Other medications like Thyroid and Anti-Diabetic drugs should be as per the Doctor's advice.

CONTRACEPTION

After delivery, the ovulation commences after a variable time. It can start as early as 4 to 6 weeks. Hence, it is important that the couple adopts some contraceptive method to prevent an unplanned pregnancy.

So, what are your options? Here's the summary.

BARRIER METHOD

Condoms are the most easily available, hence popularly used. But they are cumbersome to use and fraught with the risk of failure. There are better options.

Hormonal Injections

Normal long acting injections like DMPA can be used whose effect lasts for about three months. The dose needs to be repeated periodically. Irregular bleeding can be a bothersome side effect.

Intra Uterine Contraceptive Devices (IUCD)

The safest and the best and the most hassle free alternative is IUCD. Most commonly it is introduced by a simple OPD procedure six weeks after delivery. Various makes like Cu-T or Medicated ones like Mirena are available.

Sterilization procedures

The mother can undergo a permanent sterilization procedure at the time of Cesarean section or immediately after a normal delivery.

Laparoscopic sterilization(Lapster) is performed after six weeks or thereafter. It prevents a scar as it is done through the belly button.

Vasectomy

The surgical operation in males is easier as compared to the one in females. It is done under local anaesthesia and is almost without a scar.

It does not decrease the sexual performance or gratification in any way, as commonly believed.

WHEN SHOULD I PLAN MY NEXT PREGNANCY?

There should be at least two years gap in between the pregnancies. That allows optimum recovery of the mother as well as gives adequate time to look after the baby.

In case of Cesarean sections also, the recommendation remains the same. Contraception should be used to prevent pregnancies immediately after delivery.

Abortions should be avoided as they are fraught with their own risks.